I0411939

Book 1

Natural Homemade Cleaning Recipes for Beginners
BY LINDSEY P

&

Book 2

Soap Making For Beginners
BY LINDSEY P

Book 1

Natural Homemade Cleaning Recipes for Beginners

BY LINDSEY P

Essential Oil Recipes for Household Cleaning, Laundry & Toxic Free Living

2nd Edition

Essential Oils Box Set #29: Natural Homemade Cleaning Recipes for Beginners & Soap Making For Beginners

Table Of Contents

Introduction

I want to thank you and congratulate you for purchasing the book, *"Natural Homemade Cleaning Recipes For Beginners: Essential Oil Recipes For Household Cleaning, Laundry & Toxic Free Living"*.

This book contains proven steps and strategies on how to use essential oils to make homemade cleansers and other preparations for every part of your home. With these tips, not only will you avoid toxic substances found in commercial household cleansers, you will also save money in the long run since essential oils can be used for a variety of purposes.

Thanks again for purchasing this book, I hope you enjoy it!

Chapter 1 – Using Essential Oils

Essential oils are the distilled essences of various plants. Technically speaking, though they are called oils, they are not the same as the usual oils we use for cooking or for cosmetics. These oils are extracted from seeds or nuts, but essential oils can be extracted from other parts of the plant like the leaves, stems and even the roots. Occasionally, they are extracted from the whole plant. They are considered 'oils' because they are hydrophobic, i.e. they do not mix with water. However, they can vary in color and viscosity. Some essential oils can be clear and feel like water while some can be opaque and quite thick.

Essential oils have long been used for medicinal and cosmetic purposes, but a more common use for them has always been aromatherapy or the inhalation of their scent to create a better mood. It is common for people who would never think of lavender as a medicine or cosmetic to use it to alleviate stress. Fortunately, the spread of resources which teach people how to use essential oils for a variety of purposes has influenced more people to try more natural means for improving their well-being.

The rising trend for the use of essential oils sometimes extends to various uses in the household; but this still remains uncommon even amongst those who already use essential oils for other purposes probably because there are so many cheap household cleansers which already do a decent job. However, though these commercial products clean well enough, they are full of dangerous chemicals which can, in the long run, affect our health. Those with young children or with family members with sensitive skins and noses are most likely affected. Thus, some families are trying to search for more natural and less toxic alternatives.

While one reason some families insist on using commercial cleansers over natural cleansers with essential oils is the former is cheaper, the latter can turn out to be cheap too if all possible uses for one small bottle of essential oil are considered. Take for example lavender essential oil which many experts consider to be the most versatile. Its most obvious use is for aromatherapy to reduce stress, but it can also be used to cure acne, dandruff, psoriasis, eczema and fungal infections. It can be used to prevent and reduce fine lines and wrinkles. It can be added to natural body lotions for a relaxing scent.

For the household, it can be used to scent laundry, to sanitize surfaces and to deodorize the air. You can even cook with lavender essential oil. There are many recipes for sophisticated desserts like ice creams, cakes and jams using lavender essential oil. You can also use this to perfume soaps and shampoos.

The point being made here is one bottle of lavender essential oil can be used for a variety of purposes. Instead of buying various formulations for the purposes mentioned above, you can just buy one bottle of essential oil. Also, since essential oils are concentrated, you only need to use a small amount. Thus, one 30 ml bottle can last for months depending on how many purposes you use it for.

Buying and Safety

When using essential oils, you need to take note of one very important thing: buy true essential oil instead of artificial fragrance oil. The latter are made from artificial scents and will not give you the benefits of true essential oil other than the scent. The scent may even be inferior compared to true essential oil. While you may not be able to tell the difference, those who are used to the scent of true essential oil claim to notice a big difference in scent quality. Artificial fragrance oil can also irritate sensitive skins. If used for the laundry, it can irritate the user's skin and can even stain the clothes.

To make sure that you are using true essential oil instead of artificial fragrance oil, you should buy from reputable sources. Also, look at the label and make sure it says 100% essential oil.

Most essential oils are sold in small, opaque bottles. It is better to buy in small quantities to ensure that the product remains fresh up to the last drop. Some essential oils, particularly the citrus ones, can last only for a year. Oils which are distilled from flowers and leaves can last up to 2 years or more, but after that they will lose their efficacy and their scent might even become unpleasant. Only the thick, brownish essential oils extracted from barks, stems or roots can last for several years.

If you are only starting to use essential oils, it is better to buy the small bottle then take note of how long it lasts. After that, you can decide if you can buy the larger quantity.

If you are going to mix essential oils with other things, e.g. when making scented laundry soap, either make a fresh batch every time you need it or keep the solution in an opaque bottle and away from the sun and heat. This is to ensure that the oils do not degrade in quality.

Lastly, this book promises to teach you how to make non-toxic cleaning solutions for various purposes; however, take note that some essential oils can be as toxic as certain chemicals. For example, tea tree oil and eucalyptus essential oil must never be ingested. Wintergreen, wormwood, and camphor must never be inhaled.

Though this sounds scary, you should not be put off by this. Many reputable sellers of essential oils do not carry the dangerous essences. If you are in doubt regarding which essential oil to get, start with the safest ones like lavender and the citrus oils. The other common essential oils like tea tree, cedar wood, sandalwood and so on whose uses we will discuss in the succeeding chapters may not be safe to ingest but at least they are safe for topical use. Beginners are always advised to start with the well-known essential oils. If you wish to try other less common essential oils, be sure to do further research about their possible side effects.

In this book, for the sake of convenience, the chapters will be divided according to each room in the house. Recipes will be listed according to the tasks done in those particular rooms.

Chapter 2 – Why Use Essential Oils?

The previous chapter already explained a few things about essential oil – but what exactly makes this a good choice as a primary cleaning agent?

Aside from the fact that they're completely natural, essential oils are incredibly flexible. This means that if you keep a pure batch in your house for cleaning reasons, there's a good chance that you might use them for other needs as well. For example, you might suddenly find yourself suffering from cold or allergies – these same versions of the oil can be used to handle the problem, removing the need to purchase any type of medication.

Other known benefits of using essential oils for your cleaning needs include but are not limited to the following:

- Long term use. With years of shelf life for essential oils, you'll find that there's really no need to use them all up before expiration.
- Incredibly inexpensive, the concentrated form of these oils means that you need to use very little in order to get excellent cleaning results. That being said, a single bottle can last you years, depending on how you intend to use it.
- Depending on how DIY you want things to be, essential oils can be extracted in your own backyard using the right tools. Later on in the book, you'll find out exactly how this can be done so that you can completely track the creation of the oil.
- There is minimal health problems associated with the oil. Most people aren't allergic to these plants and warnings are available if it's not meant for the use of children and pregnant women.
- If you have pets in the house, you'll find that these essential oils will not affect them in the least. Obviously, you'll need to store the bottles properly to prevent cats/dogs from reaching them but as ingredients for cleaning, they are perfectly safe to use.

With essential oils, you are also free to experiment. You'll find that in the later chapters, we'll be providing you with recipes to mix your own batch of cleaning supplies – but you have full control over the ratio of the ingredients. If you find yourself unhappy with the results, you can experiment by adding more or subtracting some materials from the mix, creating your personal blend! For those who prefer specific scents and smells, you'll find that once you've familiarized yourself with essential oils, then you'll be able to create a mix that appeals best to your sense of smell.

Basic Essential Oils

There are literally dozens of possible essential oils out in the market today and we really can't expect you to buy each and every one of them when creating your mixes. Hence, we've narrowed down the top 10 essential oils you'll find in the market today and their important properties. You'll find that when going shopping, these are the only 10 essential oils you'll really need and they'd basically work as substitutes for oils you can't find or don't have. That being said, here's rundown of the basic essential oils every household should have:

1. **Lavender** – it is often said that if you're going to keep just one essential oil in your home, make it lavender. An all-around oil, lavender helps ease anxiety, prevent bouts of allergy, and even take care of insect bites. At home, you can use it to deodorize foul smell, especially if you happen to have any pets. It also works as a dishwashing soap ingredient and a perfect additive for candles.

2. **Tea Tree Oil** – almost all essential oils can be used as a component of dishwashing soap and tea tree oil is no different. Later, we'll teach you how to use this product to help keep your bathroom looking fresh and clean!

3. **Eucalyptus** – eucalyptus is best used to boost a person's mental acuity and is a well-known antiseptic. It's been known to help with runny-nose problems and has an excellent reputation when it comes to skin problems. As a cleaning agent, eucalyptus is often used to effectively remove bad smells as it lingers around the house.

4. **Peppermint** – perfect for soothing a tired throat due to coughs and cold, peppermint can also be used for tummy upsets and as a way to relax the muscles. Used correctly, it works perfectly as fluoride-free toothpaste and other home cleaning needs.

5. **Lemon Extract** – lemon has a strong acidic component that can be used to remove even the toughest stains. You'll find that this works well when cleaning the bathroom or kitchen, depending on how you prepare the mixture. Health-wise, it's perfect for helping with infections and easing sore throats and coughs.

6. **Rose** – what's great about this is that you can make your own rose extracts due to the abundance of the plant in the United States. With just a few drops, you'd be able to achieve excellent cleaning results – plus your house

would smell so much better! Keep in mind though that rose shouldn't be used by pregnant women.

7. **Clary Sage** - Clary Sage is a wonderful antimicrobial essential oil that's also capable of producing a relaxing scent. In fact, it's been known to help alleviate the symptoms of depression while boosting self-esteem and mental strength. It's currently one of the most popular essential oils today as evidenced by the widespread clary sage bottled products. Widely known as a wonderful eye-cleanser, this particular oil features or may be used as a substitute for many home-cleaning DIY mixes.

8. **Ylang-Ylang** – the ylang-ylang's scent alone has been proven to help with relaxation, at the same time lowering blood pressure. It works mostly as a scent additive for cleaning supplies although other use are indicated further in the book.

9. **Oregano** - An incredibly powerful antibacterial essential oil, oregano also comes with a clean and distinct scent that makes it perfect for small spaces like the bathroom. It's also known for its antifungal properties which should help when cleaning typically-damp locations like the kitchen sink or the bathroom tiles.

10. **Orange** – Orange is a pretty common type of essential oil typically used to remove stains from surfaces while giving off a wonderful scent. The great thing about this is that like lemon, you can get orange from your own backyard and turn it into essential oil, therefore removing any need to pay for the commercial version. Later on in the book, you'll find out exactly how essential oils can be extracted from their plants.

Not everyone would be happy to have all these 10 essential oils in their kitchen cabinet. The later chapters can provide you with a more detailed system for choosing what essential oils to buy, therefore limiting the number of your purchases to as little as 3.

Latin Names

Keep in mind that there are so many classifications of plants today. For example, there are different types of roses available today which means that they may be used in different essential oils. If you have health problems or highly sensitive to some materials, check by determining the Latin name of the plant used in the essential oil. A good example would be eucalyptus with around 20 different types being used today as oil. E. globulus is the most common but cannot be used by someone with epilepsy or young children. E.radiata works well against infections while E.smitthi is OK for kids. By being aware of these little nuances, you'd be able to narrow down your choices much further.

Pre Cleaning Instructions

You'll find that essential oil mixes work best if you lightly clean your target surface beforehand. For example, if you're going to use it for leather, make sure all crumbs and dust have been completely removed from the area, allowing the essential oil to fully penetrate the surface. This way, the results will be maximized and you can completely enjoy the scent as it seeps into the surface.

Chapter 3 – Kitchen

In this chapter, we will focus on the cleaning tasks done in the kitchen rather than the cooking. Though essential oils can also be used in cooking, you can check out that information from other sources.

The cleaning done in the kitchen can be categorized accordingly: food, dishes and surfaces. We will discuss each in turn.

Food

Food items like fruits and vegetables must be washed thoroughly to remove any harmful microbes and parasites from the soil which may be lurking on the surface. While you can wash these items with tap water, some of you might have sensitive stomachs and need to take extra care. If so, the essential oils you can use for this purpose include the citrus oils like lemon, grapefruit and orange.

Here is a recipe for fruit and vegetable wash:

2 cups of water

2 tablespoons of lemon juice or 1 drop of lemon essential oil

2 tablespoons of baking soda

5 drops of grapefruit or orange essential oil

Mix everything in a bowl. After the initial wash with tap water to remove visible soil and other dirt from your produce, soak everything in the essential oil solution. Scrub the hardy fruits and vegetables like apples and squashes while gently rub the soft or leafy ones like tomatoes and leafy vegetables. Rinse them again in clean water before drying.

You can make more of this solution but be sure to follow the ratio of ingredients. It is better to make this solution fresh as you need it since citrus oils are very volatile and easily lose efficacy once they are poured out of the bottle.

Long Fruit Life

Love fruits but having a hard time keeping them fresh? Put some water in a basin and put in around 5 drops of lemon essential oil. Put the fruits inside and start stirring them there for a few minutes. These fruits will last longer while ensuring that they remain as delicious and as nutritious as ever!

Trash Can Odor

Make your trash can smell good by dropping any type of citrus essential oil in a ball of cotton. Put this cotton at the bottom of the trash can and proceed as usual. The odor becomes less pungent plus it halts the development of bacteria.

Deodorize the Kitchen

Did you just cook something that doesn't really smell good? Perhaps you just cleaned the freezer or some food went bad that you weren't able to address immediately? Deal with this problem by boiling some water and adding a few drops of lavender or lemon essential oil into the mix. This will automatically dispel the bad odor in the kitchen – even reaching towards all other parts of the house.

Dishes

You can make your own dishwashing soap from diluted liquid castile soap and essential oils. Castile soap is made exclusively from vegetable oils making it very gentle to the skin. The best and most expensive varieties are made with pure olive oil, but don't discredit those made with the cheaper vegetable oils like coconut, sunflower or safflower oils since they can be good for the skin too.

Castile soap can be bought in either liquid or solid form. If you can only find solid soap, you can turn it into a liquid by grating it and dissolving the soap in an equal amount of hot water. You might wish to buy the largest quantity of castile soap you can find since this can be used for a variety of other purposes like washing clothes, cleaning various surfaces and bathing pets. You can also make shampoo and body wash from this soap.

Here is a recipe for dishwashing liquid:

2 cups of liquid castile soap

½ cup water (Adjust the amount of water or soap depending on your preference or how dirty your dishes are. Too much soap can make it difficult to rinse your dishes.)

2 drops of lemon, grapefruit or orange essential oil

5 drops of your choice of essential oils to add fragrance or you can just add more of the above

Some good choices for fragrance include the following: lavender, peppermint, lemon grass, rosemary and ylang ylang. Avoid essential oils with heavy scents like frankincense and sandalwood. Also, avoid those which can be poisonous when ingested like tea tree oil and eucalyptus. Of course, you will rinse your dishes well, but just in case some dishwashing soap lingers, you want to be on the safe side. Avoid too those which can be dangerous when inhaled like wintergreen and wormwood.

This dish soap can also be used as a hand soap and for cleaning surfaces. If you need to scour pots, pans and wooden cutting boards, add a tablespoon of baking soda to each tablespoon of dishwashing liquid to make a paste. However, if you need a more heavy duty cleanser for other kitchen surfaces, follow the recipe below.

Kitchen surfaces

Sometimes, you need a scouring cleanser to cut through grease and dirt. If so, you can use baking soda which is tough enough to remove crusted food scraps but gentle enough to not scratch surfaces.

2 cups of baking soda

½ cup of your dishwashing liquid or 3 tablespoons of liquid castile soap mixed with ½ cup water

5 drops of the same essential oil you used in your dishwashing soap or 10 drops of your choice of essential oil. In this case, you can use tea tree oil to kill the bacteria on your kitchen surfaces. As usual, avoid essential oils which should not be inhaled.

Disinfectant Spray

Lemon essential oil can be used to disinfectant kitchen surfaces, the bathroom or practically anywhere else you deem dirty. Just combine the following ingredients and spray:

Lemon oil

Water

Best places to use this combination in would include the kitchen cutting board (especially if it's made of wood), doorknobs, knives, and even the spoon and fork in your home.

Stainless Steel

Do you have lots of stainless steel in the kitchen? If so, try cleaning them by rubbing a diluted form of lemon essential oil. This makes them shine like new again! Some homeowners have noticed that it can get rid of shallow scuff marks on stainless steel and other materials. Once you're done rubbing the lemon oil, use a clean piece of cloth to further polish the steel until you can practically see your own reflection on it!

Remove Grease

Use just a drop of lemon essential oil on any greasy surface and start rubbing with a clean cloth. You'll find that this miraculously removes the grease and leaves the surface looking clean and shiny!

Sticker Problems

Ever bought a new product only to become frustrated with the sticker? Usually, the sticker leaves this residue of sticky material that just can't be rubbed off from the surface. If you have this kind of problem, try putting a few drops of lemon essential oil on the sticker and rubbing it around with a cloth. After a few seconds, the sticker residues should come off completely, leaving you with a wonderfully clean surface!

Remember, you can swap and add essential oils as you like to the recipe. Check out the chart in the later chapters to find out exactly how it's done!

Chapter 4 – Bathroom

The bathroom usually needs cleansers which can remove mildew and mold as well as provide antibacterial benefits. A fresh scent is an added plus. The cleanser recipes below range from daily maintenance to heavy duty cleaning.

Daily bathroom spray

Here is a recipe for an all-purpose bathroom cleanser for relatively clean surfaces. This can be stored in a spray bottle and used daily to prevent dirt from building up. It can also provide anti-bacterial benefits.

Equal amounts of water and white vinegar

To each cup of vinegar solution, add 5 drops of lemon, grapefruit, peppermint, lavender or tea tree essential oil

Spray this daily on non-porous surfaces and leave to dry. You can also use this on shower curtains.

Heavy duty bathroom cleanser

The same kitchen cleanser described above can be used for bathroom surfaces like shower tiles, sinks and bathtubs. If you have a problem with mildew or mold, use tea tree oil. To increase the scouring power, add more baking soda to create a thicker paste.

Toilet cleanser

If you prefer to avoid bleach, you can use undiluted white vinegar mixed with your choice of essential oil. The vinegar itself will kill microbes, but you can add more anti-microbial powers to this cleanser by using lavender or tea tree oil. Use around 10 drops of essential oil per cup of white vinegar. Use the vinegar in the same way as you would use bleach.

For particularly nasty toilets which need scrubbing, add half a cup of baking soda to each cup of vinegar. I know what you're thinking: It's going to fizz. That fizz is actually good since it will break up whatever nasty stains you have in your toilet bowl. Leave this mixture to do its work, then once it stops fizzing, use a toilet brush to scrub away any remaining dirt. Flush the toilet then pour another cup of undiluted white vinegar scented with your choice of essential oil around the bowl. Leave this mixture for at least 30 minutes or possibly overnight to kill any remaining bacteria.

Toilet Bowl Cleaner

If you're not happy using vinegar, this alternative toilet bowl cleaner should work well. Make a cleaner yourself by combining ¼ cup of castile soap, around 18 ounces of water, and 4 drops each of these essential oils: lemon, lavender, and tea tree. Put them all together in a spray bottle and start spraying all over the toilet bowl. Pay particular attention to the inside of the bowl, allowing the resulting spray to settle on the surface before scrubbing them with a brush. When done, just flush the toilet and move on to other parts! Toilet bowls should be cleaned at least once a week to ensure that there wouldn't be any gross build up of anything.

Tub and Sink Cleaner

This combination would work well for bath tubs or basically any other bathroom furniture made of the same material. Just add together ½ cup of baking soda, around 12 drops of grapefruit essential oil and 12 more of tea tree essential oil. If grapefruit isn't available, you can try using lemon or even orange to complete the recipe. To use this, give your tub a preparatory cleaning before sprinkling the essential oil infused baking soda on to the surface. Leave it there for a few minutes and begin scrubbing with a brush. Rinse when you're done and be amazed at your newly cleaned tub and the enjoyable scent lingering on the surface.

Odor absorber

Let's face it. Due to the kind of activities done in the bathroom, it can get stinky at times regardless how often you clean it. Here is a recipe for an all-natural odor absorber which removes odors instead of just masking them:

A cup of baking soda

10 drops of your choice of essential oil (or a mix to create your preferred scent)

Mix everything together and place in the corner of your bathroom preferably near the toilet. Use two bowls of this stuff if you have a large bathroom.

This is also a good odor absorber for closets and bedrooms. You can also use this to easily remove foul odors from the living room or bedroom like cigarette smoke or body odor.

Hard Water Remover

Overtime, hard water can start to crust on your pipes, shower, and faucet. When this happens, try polishing the material with lemon essential oil. This effectively removes the effects of hard water, plus it would keep your bathroom smelling wonderful.

Toilet Bombs

If you're not really keen to use a toilet bowl cleaner in liquid form, you can try creating something solid that you can just drop in the water, cleaning the surface without prompting any work on your part. The beauty of these bombs is that they don't just clean; they also produce a wonderful scent that will deodorize the bathroom. Just add together 1 1/3 of baking soda and half a cup of citric acid. These two combined can be quite dangerous so make sure you're wearing a protective mask and gloves! Stir the two together while spraying some lavender, peppermint, and lemon essential oil little by little. Make sure the acid remains intact because this will be a primary cleaner when you finally drop the bomb in the toilet. Once you're done, start putting them in small containers to dry! When they're dry, it's perfectly OK to store them someplace cold and dry, to be used at least once a week!

Chapter 5 – Living Room & Bedroom

If you need to clean hard surfaces like wood, tile or marble floors, you can use the dishwashing soap described above. Avoid using baking soda on surfaces which are easily scratched. You can also use the recipe for daily bathroom spray to mop and disinfect floors and other hard surfaces. Alternatively, you can use this mixture:

To one gallon of water, add a cup of white vinegar and 20 drops of your preferred essential oil to add scent. Take note that this scent will not last. Its only purpose is to temporarily uplift your mood while cleaning and also to temporarily mask the scent of vinegar. (The vinegar scent will dissipate once your floor dries so don't worry if you'd rather not add any essential oil to your mop water.) If you wish to scent your living room, you are better off using a diffuser, room spray, scented candle or scented potpourri.

That said, if you wish to add an essential oil which will provide both mood enhancing benefits as well as leave your floor cleaner, use lavender essential oil which will reduce stress and kill germs.

Musty carpets and upholstery

To remove unpleasant odors, you can use a mixture of baking soda and essential oil, preferably tea tree or lavender since these will kill bacteria and fungi which may be the cause of the odor. You can also add any of the citrus oils to tea tree and lavender to create a fresher scent.

Follow the recipe for odor absorber described in the previous chapter then liberally sprinkle this mixture on carpets and upholstered furniture. Leave it for at least 15 minutes then vacuum to remove the baking soda.

Leather Protection

Just got some new furniture covered by leather? If so, you can protect it from future "splitting" problems through routine application of lemon essential oil. In fact, the mixture works well with all types of leather including the inside of your vehicle, the cover of a bike, and shoes!

Cigarette Smoke Spray

Does anyone in the family smoke? If the smoke tends to linger all over the house, you can try using an essential oil spray to dispel the odor. Mix tea tree, rosemary, and eucalyptus together with water. Spray in places where the cigarette smoke is most smelled.

Polishing Furniture

If you wish to make your furniture seem new again, try mixing some lemon essential oil and olive oil together before wiping it on the surfaces. This works well for wooden furniture although obviously, you can't use the same mixture for cloth upholstery.

Jewelry

Silver jewelry can be thoroughly cleaned with just lemon essential oil. You can also try using the same mixture on any silverware in your kitchen. Gold accessories may also respond to lemon for a thorough clean.

Add Anywhere

The mint smell of peppermint makes it an excellent addition to all types of essential-oil based cleaning product. You can try adding it to some of your concoction to create a more refreshing smell. Don't add it to known chemicals however since you never know what could happen!

Window Cleaner

To achieve a smudge-free clean for your glass windows, using any type of cloth is usually a bad idea. Instead, you should try using crumpled newspapers and this will ensure the removal of smudges, lint, and other marks on the surface. To create this simply, combine around 6 drops of lemon essential oil together with 2 tablespoons of vinegar. Put in around 10 ounces of water and put them all in a spray bottle. Shake your DIY window cleaner well before spraying it on the surface and using the newspaper to achieve a wonderful shine!

You can also use the following recipe as an alternative:

½ cup white vinegar

½ cup water

10 drops of your choice of citrus essential oil

Combine everything in a spray bottle and keep it in a dark place.

Floor Cleaner

It doesn't matter if your floor is made of vinyl, laminate, ceramic, hardwood, tile, or linoleum – this all-purpose cleaner would work wonderfully every time. Combine together 1 cup of white vinegar and 1 TB of castile soap with a bucket of clean water. Add 15 drops of whatever essential oil you want (lemon and lavender

21

are best), and use this concoction to clean the floor. Spread the mix around using a mop and admire the new shine and scent of your home floor!

Heavy Duty Floor Cleaning

Not happy with the results of the original floor cleaning recipe? If you're suffering from more dirt and stain problems than expected, try adding ¼ of baking soda into the original *Floor Cleaner* mix!

Vacuum Cleaner

Having problems with your vacuum? Try putting a few drops of your favorite floral scent on a piece of tissue paper and just start sucking it up using the vacuum cleaner. You'll find that this works wonderfully well in keeping your vacuum smelling great! If you don't want to waste any tissues however, just put some drops of lemon and lavender essential oil in the water tank of the vacuum and start cleaning! This doesn't just suck up all the dirt – you're also making the whole house smell better as you go!

Wood polish

Your wood furniture and trimmings can gleam beautifully with regular polishing. You will also enjoy the pleasant smell of this polish. One recipe is enough for a middle-sized piece of furniture like a side table or dining chair.

5 drops of lemon essential oil

1 tablespoon neutral smelling plant based oil, e.g. jojoba or olive oil

1 tablespoon melted beeswax

Mix everything together before the beeswax cools.

Make two batches of this and use the second batch as a lemon lip balm. Pour it into a small metal tin sanitized with hot water and let cool before using. Your friends will think it weird that you use furniture polish as lip balm (or vice versa) but this just shows how versatile natural essential oil recipes can be.

Insect repellent

If you find your house being infested with insects, it is best to do a thorough clean-up of every hidden corner. The insects may have found a hidden food source or they may have chosen to use a dark corner of your house as their new home. It is also possible that you have not cleaned your house as thoroughly as you would like.

Whatever the case, a thorough clean will allow you to discover where the insects are coming from and the reason for their population growth.

Meanwhile, you can deter the insects from multiplying or from continuing to live in your home with these all-natural insect repellents:

Insect spray 1

1 cup of water

8 drops of black pepper essential oil

10 drops of peppermint oil

Mix everything together in a spray bottle and use where you find insects crawling. Avoid using this near food items which easily absorb odors like pasta, bread and crackers, or else keep them in air tight containers until your insect problem is solved.

Insect spray 2

Follow the same recipe described above but use 10 drops of citronella and 5 drops of orange essential oil.

Insect repellent room scent

Using a diffuser or oil burner, heat equal amounts of citronella essential oil and water. This will create a strong scent which insects hate. If you dislike the scent or if it is too strong, use a face mask. Don't open the windows and doors or the scent will disperse and weaken. Be prepared to whack cockroaches and other insects as they emerge from their dark corners. This is a good way to prevent insects from settling in your house. Do this at least once a month as a preventative measure.

Insect repellent for closets

To prevent your clothes from being consumed by insects, you can make wood insect repellents. Use small blocks of wood since they absorb and hold the essential oils better than cotton or potpourri. You can use decorative wood blocks but avoid those with paint or furniture polish.

To each palm-sized piece of wood, add 5 drops of lavender, cedar wood, cinnamon, citronella, eucalyptus or your choice of citrus essential oils. Take note that the scent will permeate your clothes, so choose whatever you will not mind smelling on yourself. You also need to choose a scent which will go well with your scented laundry soap, ironing waters or personal toiletries if ever you use these things.

Mattress Odor

Getting some unpleasant smell on your mattress? Try combining some vodka and your favorite essential oil such as lavender or lemon. Sprinkle it on the mattress and just leave it there for a few hours, allowing the liquid to dry naturally. The vodka works by killing the bacteria that causes the odor while the essential oil leaves a strong and wonderful scent behind.

Porous Stone and Granite

Mix some lemon oil with base oil and use this to polish granite and any other porous stone in your home. The lemon is capable of cleaning and restoring the shine of the material while creating a wonderful scent inside the house.

Deodorizing Disk

If the room is constantly exposed to undesirable smell, then spraying some deodorizer every few seconds may not help at all. Instead, you can try making a deodorizing disk and putting them in the center of the room so that they can constantly give off that pleasant smell. As the name suggests, the disks are mostly solid and therefore wouldn't make a mess in the house. To do this, combine:

- Lavender essential oil
- 2 cups baking soda
- 1 cup distilled water
- Molding pan

Combine the soda and water, mixing them thoroughly until you get a thick liquid past. Start dropping around 8 drops of lavender into the mix and stir again, making sure that the oil blends thoroughly with the baking soda. Put the entire concoction in a molding pan and leave them alone for 24 to 48 hours, until the soda completely hardens. Remove them from the mold and place these aromatic solids in an open jar to keep the air fresh and clean. They would be perfect in the living room, bathroom or the baby's room to ward off those nasty diaper smells.

Chapter 6 – Laundry

For laundry purposes, it is best to avoid the dark colored essential oils like sandalwood and patchouli since these might stain certain fabrics.

Scented laundry soap

Liquid castile soap can be used for washing clothes. Use ¼ cup liquid castile soap per small load of laundry. Adjust the amount of soap depending on how soiled the clothes are. To each quarter cup of soap, add 10 drops of your choice of essential oil. Mix the essential oil with the soap before adding to the washing machine.

Brighter whites

For white clothes, add 5 drops of lavender and 5 drops of lemon essential oils to each quarter cup of soap.

Stink eliminator

For foul smelling gym shirts, socks and underwear, add 5 drops of eucalyptus, 5 drops of lavender and 5 drops of tea tree oil. The 15 drops of essential oil used here will create very fragrant laundry soap, but this is necessary to neutralize the odor. This combination will also kill germs and prevent the spread of fungi.

If someone in your family suffers from fungal infections, wash his clothes separately using this laundry soap.

Fabric Softener

The great thing about using essential oil as your fabric conditioner is that you can also impart a pleasant and lasting scent on the fabric. Just dissolve around 2 tablespoons of baking soda in a ½ cup of vinegar. Add ½ teaspoon of lavender oil and pour the entire contents in the last cycle of your wash. You can also do this during the drying process by sprinkling a few drops of the oil on a dryer bowl as the clothes go through the cooling cycle.

Stain removal

Here are some tried and tested solutions to common laundry stains:

Yellow deodorant stains – soak the shirt in white vinegar and lemon essential oil. Use 5 drops of essential oil to 1 cup of vinegar.

Grease and grime – dab pure eucalyptus essential oil onto the stained parts and let it soak for at least 15 minutes before adding to the wash.

Homemade dryer sheets

For this, use one dry sock or small wash cloth for each small load of laundry. Put 5 to 10 drops of your choice of essential oil directly to the sock or wash cloth and toss this into the dryer. Add more drops for larger loads.

Washing machine disinfectant

Once in a while, run your empty washing machine with this solution: 1 cup baking soda and 10 drops of either lavender or tea tree oil. Fill the machine with water and allow it to go through a normal wash cycle. Rinse the machine well afterwards. If you wish, add another 10 drops of essential oil to the water used for rinsing.

Doing this at least once a month will ensure that your laundry will not be a breeding ground for bacteria, fungi and other germs. It is a good idea to do this after washing the clothes of an invalid or someone with a fungal infection.

Scented linen water

To add even more fragrance to your clothes, use a linen spray while ironing. Here's the recipe:

1 cup distilled water

1 tablespoon denatured alcohol or 100 proof vodka

30 drops of your preferred essential oil or a combination to create your preferred scent

Combine everything in a spray bottle and shake well. Shake the bottle before use and keep it in a cool, dark place.

This is actually a multi-purpose spray. You can also use this as a refreshing body spritz during hot days. Spray it away from the eyes and make sure you do a skin test first if you have sensitive skin. You can also use this as a room spray. Spray it on furniture, pillows and curtains to make the scent last longer. Take note that this mixture is flammable so avoid spraying it in the direction of lighted candles or light bulbs which have been on for some time.

If you are going to use scented laundry soap, dryer sheets and linen waters together, make sure that the essential oils you use go well together. You can either use just one scent for everything to play it safe, or you can combine scents. See the list below for some suggestions. Use the first for laundry soap, the second for your dryer sheet and the last for linen waters.

Ultra girly: lavender, rose, jasmine

Refreshing citrus: lemon, grapefruit, orange

Earthy herbs: lemon, rosemary, peppermint

Lemony calmer: lemon, lemon grass, chamomile

Body odor buster: lavender, tea tree oil, peppermint

Uplifting mint: eucalyptus, peppermint, peppermint or spearmint

Clothing Stain Removal

There's no need to create a mixture – just drop some lemon essential oil directly on a stain and allow it to dry for a few minutes. After that, just dump it in the washer and by the time you're done, the stain is completely removed! The great thing about this technique is that it works on practically all types of fabric,

Cleaning Cloth Diapers

Cloth diapers are wonderfully inexpensive and perfect if your child has sensitive skin. To make it more effective however, try adding around 5 drops of tea tree oil in your washing detergent. You can also soak the cloth diapers in water first and add the tea tree oil in this stage. An excellent antimicrobial product, this ensures that your child wouldn't be exposed to any germs while wearing the diaper.

Pine Gum and Tree Sap

If you ever find yourself having problems with pine gum on your clothes, try using pure lemon oil to remove the stain. You can also remove chewing gum using the same mixture. This works well and provides an excellent smell to the clothing.

Chapter 7 – Plants, Pets, Pests, and Personal

The last household use for essential oils is for the removal of pests from your house plants and pets.

Plants

To prevent house plants from being destroyed by insects and other small creatures, you can follow these recipes:

Anti-aphid and ant plant spray

5 drops of spearmint essential oil

7 drops of orange or lemon essential oil

1 quart of water

2 tablespoons salt

Mix everything in a spray bottle and spray directly onto the plant.

Anti-snail solution

Use wooden disposable chopsticks or bamboo skewers. Add a few drops of patchouli, cedar wood or sandalwood essential oil to each. Stick them near the plants which have been plagued by snails. Reapply oils once the scent dissipates.

Anti-beetle solution

Use the same method described above but use peppermint, lemongrass or thyme essential oil.

Anti-slug solution

Use the same method described above but use cedar wood or pine essential oil.

Pets

For pets, you can use essential oils to minimize odor, prevent and kill fleas and ticks, and also for aromatherapy.

Anti-odor dog shampoo 1

Use liquid castile soap as a shampoo. Start with 2 tablespoons of soap for a medium-sized dog such as a cocker spaniel then add more depending on how dirty your pet is. To each tablespoon of soap used, add 1 to 2 drops of tea tree oil to prevent odors and to help prevent fleas and ticks.

Anti-odor dog shampoo 2

If you ran out of castile soap, you can use baking soda. This is a cheaper alternative which can be a better choice if you have a lot of dogs and don't want to spend too much on castile soap. This is also a better choice for smellier dogs.

Dissolve ½ cup of baking soda in ½ cup of water to make a paste. To each cup of paste, mix in 1 to 2 drops of tea tree oil.

Anti-odor pet powder

In between baths, use baking soda mixed with lavender or tea tree oil to prevent nasty odors from forming. Use about 5 drops of essential oil per half cup of baking soda. You can also sprinkle this mixture onto your pet's beddings.

Flea and tick spray

Tea tree oil is great for preventing and killing fleas and ticks. Mix 10 drops of the essential oil in 1 cup of water and spray liberally. Avoid spraying your pet's face. Alternatives can be peppermint, oregano, thyme or cinnamon.

Flea and tick powder

As an alternative to the above, you can combine 5 drops of the recommended essential oils to ½ cup of baking soda and use this to prevent fleas and ticks. The baking soda will also minimize odor.

Fly Repellent

To keep flies from flying in and settling in your home, try making a spray containing lavender. Add around 25 drops of the essential oil with 16 ounces of water and shake well. You can start spraying this all over the house, especially in places where flies are more likely to settle. This would work wonderfully for the kitchen plus you'd be able to enjoy the pleasant odor.

Pet aromatherapy

Believe it or not, aromatherapy can also work for pets. You need to use a weaker scent for animals, especially for dogs, since they have heightened scent glands. You can use a diffuser, oil burner, scented candle or room spray. You can also add a few drops of essential oil to a cotton ball and tape it above your pet's cage or bed. Do not spray your pet with scented body sprays which contain alcohol since this might irritate their skin.

Calming

If your pet exhibits signs of nervousness or agitation, use lavender to calm it down. This is also a good choice to make newly bought pets feel at home.

Increase concentration

If you are training your pet, use peppermint, jasmine or grapefruit.

Pest Prevention

If you constantly have problems with mice, squirrel, and even spiders – a few drops of peppermint will work wonders. Just put a few drops in a cotton ball and place them in likely places the pests use to move in and out of the house.

Personal Soap

Since you're cleaning your home using essential oils, you might as well extend this to your personal hygiene. Fortunately, making soap is easy enough to do – plus you can choose whatever scent you want. There are lots of recipes online if you want to start from scratch. If you want an easier way of doing this however, just grab some basic liquid castile soap and drop some essential oil into the mix to create that wonderful scent. The beauty of castile soap is that not only is it cheap – it also works for all parts of the body and rarely triggers any skin problems.

For instructions on personal soap making, here's a good recipe that lets you cook your own without handling chemicals:

- 500g Melt and pour soap
- Mold
- Heatproof jug
- Microwave oven
- At least 3 essential oils
- Rubbing alcohol fine spray

Step 1 – start cutting or shredding the melt and pour soap into tiny pieces so it would melt faster. A 500g melt and pour should make around 3 to 4 bars.

Step 2 – put the shredded pieces in the microwave and heat it up for 1 minute. Open the door and check if it has fully melted. If not, shut the microwave and turn it on again for 15 seconds. Do this repeatedly until you get the liquid consistency you want. Note that putting it inside for more than 60 seconds can damage the soap.

Step 3 – remove the soap from the microwave, being very careful because of the heat. Start stirring the soap, making sure that no skin will form at the top. This is also the time to add your favored essential oils. Mix thoroughly to ensure that the scent clings to the soap.

Step 4 – quickly pour the liquid soap in the mold and allow it to chill. You can try tapping the mold several times in the event of any air bubbles. This way, you can be sure that every pocket of air is fully filled with the soap. Leave it to harden in open air or put it in the fridge for faster results.

Putting color in your soap is also a good idea, but make sure to find soap-friendly dye. Note though that the color doesn't really add anything to the soap but only offers aesthetic benefits. Other ingredients like oatmeal and honey also work wonderfully well in adding to the quality of the product. You'll find that with this, you can save a lot in the process! Some combinations you can try out:

- Bergamot, lime, orange, and lemon
- Oakmoss, courmain, and lavender
- Vanilla, cinnamon, and tonka bean
- Helional, violet, leaf, and estrogen
- Eroli, ylang-ylang, black pepper, and jasmine

Personal Shampoo

Having a hard time finding the perfect shampoo for your hair? Perhaps it's time to make your own! Here are the instructions for a DIY personal shampoo with essential oil additions!

- Half a cup of liquid castile soap
- ¼ cup of honey
- ¼ cup of canned coconut milk
- 1 tbsp vitamin-e oil
- 50 drops of your favored essential oil or a combination of many
- 2 tbsp of fractioned coconut oil

Step 1 – Mix all the above ingredients together using an empty bottle of shampoo or any other container you can find. Make it is thoroughly shaken instead of just being mixed with an apparatus.

Step 2 – put in a container of your choice and use it like regular shampoo! You can try adding more stuff if you want, depending on how your hair reacts to the basic recipe.

Step 3 – shake the bottle before every use to make sure you can benefit from all the ingredients with every drop!

Step 4 – make just enough of the shampoo to be used within one month. It can be problematic if the item is stored for longer periods of time. Like commercial shampoo, try not to put the item in direct sunlight or anywhere heated.

Dandruff Problems – if you have dandruff problems, aim for a mix containing a mix of lemon, rosemary, melaleuca, and lavender. All these work together to stop dandruff, nourish your hair and provide excellent smell at the same time.

Hair Loss – a shampoo that addresses this problem should contain the following essential oils: rosemary, cedarwood, peppermint, and lavender.

Damaged and Fragile Hair – Lavender, clary sage, and wild orange work best if you love to style and color your hair, resulting to damage.

Body Splash

This invigorating mix can be an excellent addition to your personal care collection!

- 4 ½ teaspoon of vodka
- 18 drops of essential oils
- 2 tsp distilled water

Combine all the ingredients and store them in a glass and dark container for two weeks. Shake them as often as possible during those two weeks to completely combine the oils together. After the requisite 14 days, filter the mixture through a coffee filter before placing in your fine mist bottle. Enjoy the new scent and make bigger batches once you're happy with the results!

Chapter 8 – Essential Oil Swapping Chart and Scents

In the previous Chapters, we've given you several recipes to help with cleaning, but what if you can't find the specific essential oil you need as indicated in the recipe? Fortunately, it's perfectly OK to swap essential oils as long as you know exactly what their properties are. Most essential oils fall within specific categories and should you have any problem finding say, eucalyptus essential oil, there are several other types that you can use as a substitute. Here's a chart that would help.

CATEGORY	WHAT IT DOES	ESSENTIAL OIL
Antimicrobial	As the name suggests, these oils offer excellent cleaning benefits in the sense that they remove traces of microbes on the surface. This makes them perfect for the bathroom, kitchen, and anywhere where germs are most likely to spread	• Tea tree oil (also antifungal) • Peppermint • Clary sage • Lemon • Lavender • Oregano (powerful)
Citrus	Essential oils coming from the citrus family are usually added in for their fresh and clean scent. You'll find that many commercial products utilize citrus in their ingredients to mask the smell of chemicals. What you should know however is that it also works wonderfully for removing stains. The slightly acidic element of citrus makes it an excellent choice if you want to remove marks from the surface of furniture, clothes, and even dishes.	• Lemon • Tangerine • Orange • Spearmint • Grapefruit
Floral	These are basically essential oils contributing mostly 'scent' to the cleaning mix. Although they also have unique cleaning properties, these are mostly added for their wonderful aroma	• Rose • Ylang-ylang • Neroli • Jasmine
Minty	Contributes mostly to scent	• Peppermint • Spearmint

Woodsy	Contributes mostly to scent	• Pine • Cedar
Oriental	Contributes mostly to scent	• Ginger • Patchouli
Earthy	Contributes mostly to scent	• Oakmoss • Vetiver • Patchouli
Herbaceous	Contributes mostly to scent	• Marjoram • Basil • Rosemary
Spicy	Contributes mostly to scent	• Nutmeg • Cinnamon • Clove

Perfect Blending Options

All essential oils blend well together, but it might take some time before you hit the exact smell you want. Here's a guide that could help you get started:

- Floral works well with anything citrus, woodsy, or spicy
- If you like oriental, you can blend it with something spicy and add a few drops of floral or citrus
- Mints works well with herbaceous, citrus and woodsy

Experiment as much as you want and have fun!

Essential Oil Notes

This refers to how long a scent lasts depending on the note of the essential oil. Top notes usually evaporate faster and therefore lose their scent faster. Base notes however last the longest. Here's a chart of the different notes and the oils that fall under them. Use this information when making your own blends for house or personal hygiene.

TOP	BASE	MIDDLE
Orange	Ginger	Rose
Lemon	Beeswax	Ylang-ylang

Essential Oils Box Set #29: Natural Homemade Cleaning Recipes for Beginners & Soap Making For Beginners

Lemongrass	Vanilla	Parsley
Peppermint	Angelica Root	Nutmeg
Tangerine	Myrrh	Cypress
Lavender	Oakmoss	Cinnamon
Lime	Cedarwood	Clary Sage
Eucalyptus	Sandalwood	Bay
Bergamot	Patchouli	Black Pepper

When mixing practically anything using essential oils, it would also work best to combine a Top, Middle, and Base note in the mixture. This is especially true if you're using essential oils primarily for their wonderful smell.

The Scents and Moods

You might also want to consider the activity in each room before choosing what essential oil to use in the area. With these oils typically used in aromatherapy to create a "mood", you'll find that using them in specific parts of the house can enhance your enjoyment of the room. Take the following for example:

Clean and Invigorating Scent

The living room and kitchen can be the site of much traffic and activity in the house. If you want to promote a lively feeling within this room, try using the following essential oils in your cleaning mix: peppermint, grapefruit, ylang-ylang, chamomile and lemon.

Relaxing Scents

Having trouble sleeping? There are lots of essential oils that can help you achieve a relaxed and therefore sleepy mood. Try using chamomile, bergamot, clary sage, cedarwood, jasmine, lavender, rose, ylang-ylang, jasmine, and geranium in your bedroom cleaning mixtures. You can also try adding them in your DIY fabric softener when washing the sheets and pillow covers. This way, you'd be able to lie right on top of the smell's source, giving you a wonderful night's sleep.

Enhances Concentration

The library, computer room, mini-office or even the kid's study desk can be polished by mixtures enhanced by lavender essential oil. Studies show that this particular scent can help individuals with their focus, boosting concentration and essentially helping with productivity. If lavender isn't available, you can also use peppermint, cinnamon, ginger, and sage.

WRITE IT DOWN!

When making a personal blend, it's usually a good idea to write down the progress you're making. It's incredibly easy to lose track of how many drops you're adding to the mix so make sure every drop is accounted for. Try using a cotton ball for the mixture and time how long before the scent starts to disappear. Note that although essential oils can be calming, prolonged exposure to a consistently strong scent can induce headaches. Hence, only play with the oils for short periods of time – remember, it's a hobby!

Once you're more aware of what essentials oils can do, you'll be able to create personalized cleaning solutions that suit your needs and scent preferences. Keep in mind though that the quality of the essential oil plays an important role in the end-results of your mix. Refer to Chapter 1 to find out exactly how to buy your essential oil ingredients.

Chapter 9 – DIY Essential Oil Extraction & FAQ

If you'll notice, most of the essential oils provided here are pretty common in their plant form. Oregano, rose, peppermint, orange, lemon, and others can be grown in your own backyard year round – so why not make your own? This way, you wouldn't have to worry about the essential oils expiring because you'll only make what you need and even if they expire – there's more in the backyard!

In this Chapter, we'll teach you exactly how to extract your own essential oils:

Step 1: Purchase a Distiller

A distiller is usually your best option when making your own essential oil. This is sold few a few hundred dollars and can supply you with a fresh batch of essential oil every time you need them. Of course, you can also make your own, utilizing different designs offered through the internet. Distillers typically have the same components which include: the heat source, the container, the condenser, and the separator.

Step 2: Harvest with Care

Start harvesting the plants you need, being very careful in the process. You don't want these plants crushed or torn because this can affect the quality of the essential oil. As much as possible, extract the oil on the same day as you harvested the plant to ensure that you get only the best portions for your oil. If you're going to purchase the plants, make sure to get them from a reliable source and asking when they were harvested. Steer clear of powdered portions of the plant.

Step 3: Start Cooking!

If you're using a commercial distiller, follow the instructions as listed down by the manufacturer. This includes the amount of the water that should be put in the tank as well the ideal length of time for distillation. Typical essential oil extraction procedures require that the plant should NOT be touching the water. For hydro distillation however, you'd want the plants to be floating on the water. Cooking time may be anywhere from one to six hours, depending on the plant you have and manufacturer instructions. In most cases, you only need to boil the water once until it has completely condensed. In some instances however, you might need to refill the tank and continue with the boiling to extract as much oil as possible.

Step 4: Separate and Store

Now that you're done with the boiling process, separate the oil by using a clean cloth to squeeze them out! Make sure the cloth is clean – you don't want the essential oils contaminated by detergents used for the fabric. As for storage, it's best to keep the oil in a tightly packed container made from glass. Keep it safe in a cool place away from direct sunlight and damp.

You'll find that there's some leftover water, typically named "hydrosol". Hydrosol is basically any water left behind after you've run the plant through the separator. This also contains some of the essential elements of the plant and will work well for several maladies. You can check out how lavender water or lemon water can be used in your daily activities through the internet. It's also possible to use this water for your next distilling process IF you plan to do another one on the same day. If not, it's best to discard them properly. Don't forget to wear gloves and other protective clothing when distilling your own essentials oils since they can be hazardous when applied directly on the skin!

Frequently Asked Questions

Want to find out more about essential oils that wasn't discussed in this book? This FAQ section should help deal with any questions you might have.

I'm pregnant – can I use essential oils?

The answer to this question depends largely on how you intend to use essential oils. Are you going to ingest it, apply it topically, or just smell it? If you're pregnant, some essential oils should definitely be avoided but others are friendly enough. Some of the pregnant-friendly oils include: ylang-ylang, orange, tea tree oil, cypress, and lavender. If unsure, do not use the oil and refer to a medical professional. If you're using a commercial essential oil, the instructions at the back of the bottle should tell you the limits of its use.

What if I'm breastfeeding – can I use the oils?

Yes, but you have to choose exactly what oils you can use. Although the child isn't directly affected, some oils are remarkably strong and therefore can cause problems to the child, especially if it absorbs the oil orally through the breasts. Fortunately, there's an extensive list of breastfeeding-friendly oils, as long as you use them sparingly. This includes: geranium, lavender, lemon, sandalwood, clary sage, ylang-ylang, wild orange, and grapefruit.

Can I use essential oils on children?

Children are more susceptible to the harsh side of essential oils. When applied topically, you have to keep in mind that the skin of children is thinner and could therefore produce negative results. When diluted properly however, these same essential oils can work wonders and may be used to clean baby things. In fact, you'll find that using essential oil infused fabric softeners for your baby's clothes would work wonderfully and can even help the child sleep at night.

I though we're supposed to dilute the oil before using it?

Yes, diluting the oil is definitely necessary if you intend to apply it on the skin, inhale the mix or add it to food. Since you're using it for cleaning purposes however, an undiluted mix is best because this increases the cleaning impact of the product. Should you wish to use it for other purposes however, mixing the essential oil with carrier oil would be best. At the bottom of this chapter, we'll provide you with a Diluting Chart for Essential Oils.

Is expensive better?

Not necessarily. There are few manufacturers of essential oils today, which mean that most products probably came from the same source. Unless you plan to apply the material directly on your skin or ingest it, purchasing an inexpensive batch shouldn't be a problem. Fortunately, essential oils last long and can survive for years when stored correctly. A single bottle may serve you for a very long time since you only need a few drops of each to create a clean-worthy mixture.

Is just bought my second essential oil from the same company and it smells different!

Don't be wary – this is actually a good thing! It shows that the manufacturer is providing the purest essential oils rather than trying to add chemicals in the mix to make it more uniform. See, plant yields are never the same each time. The weather while it was growing, the soil content and various other aspects of the planting process come into play when it comes to essential oils. Hence, don't worry too much about the difference in smell because this doesn't really affect the cleaning capacity of the oil.

Should I buy bark essential oil or leaf?

You'll find that essential oils are labeled depending on which part of the plant they were taken from. Some may be derived from the bark, others from the flower while there are those taken from the bark. Aroma therapists typically prefer bark concentrations because they offer better antibacterial properties. Hence, if you want better cleaning results, utilize eucalyptus and tea tree bark essential oils since they're the ones that work best against bacteria. Everything else is left to your discretion.

Are aromatherapy oils the same thing?

Although it's true that you can use essential oils for aromatherapy, that doesn't mean that aromatherapy oils can be utilized as essential oils. The two are completely different and you shouldn't interchange their uses. Aromatherapy is far from pure, usually containing petroleum so that they can be added in candles or used for massages. Simply put, you won't be getting the same results with this one.

What about allergies?

Essential oils are basically a more potent version of the plants they came from. That being said, if you have an allergy on tea tree, there's a good chance that its oil will also have a negative effect on you. If you're not sure, dilute the oil using some carrier oil and apply it on your skin, around the inside of your wrist. Wait for 24 hours to see if there are any rashes or itchiness showing up. If not, then you're good to go and you can start using the essential oil for various home cleaning projects.

Dilution Chart

CARRIER OIL	1%	2%	3%	5%	10%
5 ML	1 drop	2 drops	3 drops	5 drops	10 drops
10 ML	2 drops	4 drops	6 drops	10 drops	20 drops
15 ML	3 drops	6 drops	9 drops	15 drops	30 drops
20 ML	4 drops	8 drops	12 drops	20 drops	40 drops

Essential Oils Box Set #29: Natural Homemade Cleaning Recipes for Beginners & Soap Making For Beginners

25 ML	5 drops	10 drops	15 drops	25 drops	50 drops

1% Dilution is best used by people with sensitive skin such as children, the elderly and pregnant women. The 2% dilution is the perfect choice for healthy adults while 10% offers a more powerful punch used for muscular pain. Just follow the chart pattern if you want to increase the dilution of your essential oils. For cleaning purposes, you can steadily increase the amount of drops added in, depending on how tough the stains and dirt happens to be. Remember – essential oils can damage plastic so don't use this when cleaning anything plastic!

Conclusion

Thank you again for purchasing this book!

I hope this book was able to help you to know how to use essential oils for various household needs.

The next step is to try out the recipes described here and choose which works for you. You don't always have to stick to these recipes. You can tweak them according to your personal preferences.

Finally, if you enjoyed this book, please take the time to share your thoughts and post a review on Amazon. We do our best to reach out to readers and provide the best value we can. Your positive review will help us achieve that. It'd be greatly appreciated!

Thank you and good luck!

Book 2

Soap Making For Beginners
BY LINDSEY P

A Guide to Making Natural Homemade Soaps from Scratch, Includes Recipes and Step by Step Processes for Making Soaps

Essential Oils Box Set #29: Natural Homemade Cleaning Recipes for Beginners & Soap Making For Beginners

Copyright 2014 by Lindsey P - All rights reserved.

Table Of Contents

Introduction

I want to thank you and congratulate you for purchasing the book, "Soap Making For Beginners: A Guide To Making Natural Homemade Soaps From Scratch, Includes Recipes and Step By Step Processes for Making Soaps."

This book contains proven steps and strategies on how to create natural homemade soaps using easy to obtain ingredients.

This book is perfect for those who want to make their own soap but do not know where to begin. Soap making is a fun and rewarding hobby that you can also turn into a business once you have successfully made your first batch of soap. In this book, you will get to know the different ingredients, tools and processes on how to create soap.

Thanks again for purchasing this book, I hope you enjoy it!

Chapter 1 - Hello, Soap Making Starter!

Making your own batch of natural soap at home has many advantages. First of all, you get to enjoy hypoallergenic soap that can even clear up facial acne and skin blemishes. The perfectly processed soap acts as a gentle cleanser and moisturizer that is fun to make and pleasurable to use.

How Soap is Formed

Soap forms when lye and water chemically react together with oil, turning the oil into a salt. This is known as "saponification." Lye should be slowly added (never poured!) into the water. Once you add the lye and water to the oil, the mixture will start to thicken, and the primary stage of this thickening is referred to as "light trace". The "gel stage" takes place once the soap becomes so heated up that it starts to look like applesauce. This is full saponification and it means that the soap is almost completely formed. It will keep on thickening until it becomes a solid bar.

There are two types of process in forming soap, and these are cold process and hot process (you will know more about them in chapter 3). It takes around 24 to 48 hours for the saponification to occur in cold process soap, while in hot process the soap will have already saponified after it is done cooking.

Solid soaps are formed with "alkalis", while liquid soap are formed with potassium hydroxide. These ingredients are dangerous if not handled properly.

You should only use pure lye that is specifically for making soap. You can buy this online or you can use Red Devil lye. If you do not want to use lye you can opt for the melt and pour soap, which is a finished soap product with directions on how to process it.

Soaps' shelf life depends a lot on their ingredients, particularly the iodine value. Some soaps can last for years, while others do not last for over twelve months. If the iodine in the soap is too high it will create what are called "dreaded orange spots" or DOS, which is a sign that the soap is stale. You will learn about how to calculate the ingredients in your soap carefully using a soap calculator (soapcalc.net), including the iodine value.

To keep soap fresh, it is recommended that you keep it in a closed plastic container such as a plastic shoe box. Soap can absorb scents quickly, and you do not want it to absorb other scents apart from the one that you used with it.

Soap Making Safety Equipment

Soap making should be done in a room wherein you will not be disturbed by your kids, visitors or pets. You will also need a few basic and inexpensive safety equipment to keep yourself safe. These are:

Gloves. You will need latex gloves like the ones being used by doctors. These are inexpensive and can be found in any drugstore.

Safety Goggles or Face Shield. Wear a pair of safety goggles that are resistant to heat and will wrap around your eyes completely. If you wear glasses, then you can opt for the full face shield instead. Both are relatively inexpensive and can be found in any hardware store.

Long-sleeved Shirt and Apron. You will need to protect your skin and clothes from lye and potassium hydroxide for these can irritate the skin and burn a hole upon contact on your clothing.

Shoes. Always wear shoes - never wear slippers, sandals nor go barefoot - while making soap. Any spills or splatters will burn your skin. Wear a pair of closed shoes which you won't mind getting splattered on.

Vinegar. This is more of a first aid item that you need to have at hand because it neutralizes lye. If any lye splatters onto your skin, immediately wash it off with water and pour vinegar onto it to remove all traces.

In the next chapter, you will get to know the different basic ingredients and tools that you will need in making natural soap.

Chapter 2 - Get to Know the Basic Tools and Ingredients of Soap Making

In preparing for soap making, make sure that the venue is off limits to other people, especially kids and pets. After all, you do not want to risk any injuries. Now let's jump right into the list of tools and ingredients that you will need for your soap making project.

Basic Tools

The tools that you will need in making soap are inexpensive and easy to obtain. These are:

Handheld immersion blender. This type of blender is sticklike with a spinning blade on one end. This is used mostly for drinks or whipping cream but in this case you will be using it for making soap. It helps minimize the energy spent on stirring but you can skip this if your arm is used to stirring for extended periods of time.

Stainless steel stockpot with lid. If you already have one in your kitchen you can use that. It needs to be very clean and still be safe enough to cook food in. Ideally, it should hold from three to twelve quarts to create a nice batch of soap. Never use aluminum or enamel-ware pots because the lye will eat through these types of material.

Bowls. Use only plastic or stainless steel bowls while measuring your soap ingredients. You can also use a plastic pitcher (never glass!) that has a lid to mix lye.

Whisk or spoon and Spatula. Only use a whisk or spoon made of stainless steel or the kind made for using with nonstick pans. Do not use wooden.

Scale. You will need a quality electronic kitchen scale with a platform that can any of the bowls and pitchers that you will be using. It should measure to 1/10 an ounce and should also measure in grams.

Stainless steel thermometer. You will need this to check the oils', lye and water temperature to find out the right time to mix the oils with the lye and water. If you do not have a thermometer, you can touch the outside of the pitcher or pot using your fingers. You will know when the lye and water can be added to the oil once the heat is bearable to the touch.

Soap Molds. Any container except metal can be used as a soap mold. Some suggestions would be plastic tray molds with cute designs on top. A 5x6 inch container can hold 1.5 pounds or 24 ounces of soap. There are plenty of wooden, acrylic and plastic soap molds that you can shop for online with a wide variety of designs to choose from.

Basic Ingredients

You do not need a lot of ingredients to create a simple bar of natural soap. Here is an overview:

Oils and butters. These work as the bases of the soap. The different oils and butters have varied properties with specific uses. Base oils are palm oil, lard and tallow. Cleansing oils are palm kernel, babassu, and coconut oil. For lather and moisturizing, use Castor oil.

Lye. You cannot make soap without lye. Sodium hydroxide is used for creating solid (bar) soap while potassium hydroxide is used for creating liquid soap. Lye produces a toxic vapor when it is added and stirred into the water. Make sure that your room is well-ventilated and you are wearing a protective mask.

Borax. This ingredient is needed to neutralize the leftover lye in liquid soap, lower the pH, and improve its cleaning power. It is also a deodorizer and disinfectant.

Additives

Naturally you would want your soap to be a lot more fun than just the basic bar. There are plenty of additives that you can incorporate into your soap mixture such as fragrance, milk, honey, herbs and so on.

If you wish to use fragrance oils, use only those that are guaranteed safe for the skin. Essential oils can be used but must be at a minimum (about a maximum of 2.5 percent) because too much of this can irritate the skin.

You can also use liquid colorants to make you soap look more attractive. Just make sure to use the kind that is safe on the skin such as micas or oxides.

Choosing Oils and Butters

As a soap making starter, shea butter is an excellent type of butter that is great for soap making. It has moisturizing properties that can also increase lather. Three basic oils for soap making are coconut oil, castor oil, and palm oil.

There are plenty of other oils and butters that you can use for soap making as well. Here is a list:

- Almond Oil

- Apricot Kernel Oil

- Avocado Oil

Essential Oils Box Set #29: Natural Homemade Cleaning Recipes for Beginners & Soap Making For Beginners

- Babassu Oil
- Canola Oil
- Castor Oil
- Cocoa Butter
- Corn Oil
- Emu Oil
- Flaxseed Oil
- Grapeseed Oil
- Hemp Seed Oil
- Illipe Butter
- Jojoba Oil
- Karanja Oil
- Kokum Butter
- Lanolin
- Lard
- Mango Butter
- Mowrah Butter
- Neem Seed Oil
- Olive Oil
- Olive Oil Pomace
- Ostrich Oil
- Palm Oil
- Palm Kernel Oil
- Peanut Oil
- Rice Bran Oil
- Safflower Oil (High Oleic)
- Sal Butter

- Shea Butter

- Soybean Oil

- Sunflower Oil (High Oleic)

- Beef Tallow

Do some more research on each oil and butter on your own and you will find an encyclopedia of benefits along with specific properties. Most of these oils and butters can be bought in your local grocery store.

Fragrances

To add scent to your soap, you can make use of fragrances or essential oils. Fragrance oils are synthetic blends made up of chemicals that copy the scents of essential oils. Below is a list of the most commonly used fragrances:

- Spellbound Woods

- Black Tea and Berries

- Cool Mountain Lake

- Lavender Rose

- Cucumber Mint

- Hardwood Musk

- Fresh Pomegranate

Keep in mind that there are close to 8,000 fragrances available on the market. Have fun trying them all! Just make sure to use skin-safe and avoid the ones containing the chemical called "phthalates" because these are harmful to your skin. Opt for higher quality oils because the scent will last much longer even if they are more expensive. You can use about .5 to .7 ounce of strong fragrance oil per pound of oil compared to using 1 ounce per pound of oil if you use cheaper fragrance oil.

Essential Oils

Essential oils do not just smell good but they also have medicinal properties. They are distilled from bark, flower, roots, stems or leaves of plants and can be too potent, so use sparingly. Here is a list of essential oils commonly used in soap making:

- Balsam Peru

**Essential Oils Box Set #29: Natural Homemade Cleaning Recipes for Beginners &
Soap Making For Beginners**

- Sweet Basil

- Bay laurel

- Bay rum

- Benzoin

- Bergamot

- Cajeput

- Carrot Seed

- Cedarwood, atlas

- Cinnamon bark

- Clary sage

- Combava petitgrain

- Coriander

- Cypress

- Elemi

- Eucalyptus

- Eucalyptus, lemon

- Fir Needle

- Frankincense

- Geranium

- Grapefruit, pink

- Jasmine

- Juniper berry

- Lavender

- Lemongrass

- Manuka

- Myrrh

- Myrtle

- Neroli
- Niaouli
- Oak moss absolute
- Bitter Orange
- Oregano
- Patchouli
- Peppermint
- Rosalina
- Rosemary
- Rosewood
- Sage
- Spearmint
- Spikenard
- Spruce
- Stryax resin
- Tangerine
- Tea tree
- Thyme
- Verbena
- Vetiver, El Salvador
- Violet leaf
- Yarrow
- Ylang ylang

Do extensive research on each essential oil and you will find a wide range of medicinal benefits. Many of these essential oils have natural antibacterial properties. Just make sure not to use peppermint essential oil on diabetics and be careful in selecting the right essential oils for infants younger than 3 months as well as pregnant women. You can blend your essential oils and be as creative as you like.

Chapter 3 - Soap Making Made Easy by SoapCalc

Soon you will get to know the basic steps on how to process soap. There are mainly two basic processes, the Hot Process and Cold Process. But before moving on to these two, let's first discuss a very useful online tool that you can use in formulating the perfect soap recipes.

Using SoapCalc

It is very easy to formulate the kind of soap that you would like to create. All you will need is a computer or Smart Phone and internet connection. Visit www.soapcalc.net and all of the instructions will be given to you there.

In SoapCalc, all you have to do is to type in the ingredients and to pick the qualities that you would like for your soap. After clicking a button, SoapCalc will give you the recipe and recommendations on the right amount of water and lye that you will need to get the recipe that you want..

If it all seems too confusing at first, you can start practicing with this basic soap recipe:

Basic soap is made up of 70 percent Palm oil, 20 percent coconut oil, and 10 percent castor oil.

Step 1: in Box 2 in soapcalc.net, click on the "Ounces" button (box 6 will change to "oz.") and type in "11".

Step 2: in Box 3, convert the "Water as % of Oils" from default (which is 38 percent) to 30.

Step 3: in Box 4, convert the "Super Fat %" to "10", and for fragrance, type ".5".

Step 4: In the list of oils, double click on "Palm". Click the circle over the "%" and the column will turn green. Type in "70" beside Palm.

Step 5: Double click on "Coconut (76 deg, solid) and then, in the green field beneath %, type in "20".

Step 6: Double click "Castor Oil" and add "10" in the green field.

Step 7: In Box 8, click the "Calculate Recipe".

If you do not get 100 percent, you will see a pop-up box that will show how much you need to add or subtract in order to get 100 percent.

You will see a "View or Print Recipe" button. Once you click it, you will see your soap recipe in a new window.

**Essential Oils Box Set #29: Natural Homemade Cleaning Recipes for Beginners &
Soap Making For Beginners**

Find the time to explore soapcalc.net in order to familiarize yourself with its features. Once you start working on your own first batch of soap, you are most likely to be successful while using this tool.

Chapter 4 - Cold Process Soap

Cold Process or CP soap is when the saponification happens while the mixture is in the mold. It takes longer for the soap to cure this way compared to the Hot Process. "Curing" is the state wherein the water evaporates and the soap would harden.

The first part of the process is to mix fixed oils (such as Palm, Coconut or Olive) with alkali (lye or Sodium hydroxide). After that you bring the batch to trace. "Trace" is the state wherein the soap batch thickens. There are 3 trace stages, and these are light, medium, and thick. The moment trace begins, you will notice a ripple when you check the back of your spoon or immersion blender while you move it through the mixture. Light trace will have the consistency of thin sauce. Medium trace has the consistency of gravy. Thick trace will be similar to a pudding.

Once it is in the Medium stage of trace, you pour the mixture into the mold and use wax paper to cover it. Finally, you set it aside to solidify.

Cold process soap will have a texture that is creamier compared to hot process soap. Choosing this process will also enable you to be in complete control over the ingredients. Most often, the soaps will have a longer shelf life as well. One disadvantage is that it takes from four to six weeks of curing time. Because of this, some essential oils and fragrance oils do not outlast the cold process and would undergo chemical decomposition.

Cold Process Oven Process. A modified CP method called the Cold Process Oven Process or CPOP method is a great way to reap the benefits of CP soap without the extended waiting time. Certain batches can cure for only two or three days. The only change that you need to do in the cold process soap instructions is to not just set the soap-filled mold aside, but to put it in the oven.

Right before mixing the ingredients, preheat your oven to 170 degrees Fahrenheit (76.67 degrees Celsius). After you have mixed the lye and oils and poured it into the mold, cover it with wax paper. Next, you turn off the oven but keep the oven light on. After that, you place the mold into the oven and let it sit there for a few hours to cool. Remove the soap once it is hard enough and cut into bars. After that, let it sit for a few more days.

It is ideal to let the soap sit for 48 hours before the soap is taken out of the mold and set on a drying rack. The soap should be left to dry for another 24 to 48 hours before it is cut into bars. Soap is typically cut at 3.25 inches in length and 2.25 inches in width.

How to Make Cold Process Soap

Essential Oils Box Set #29: Natural Homemade Cleaning Recipes for Beginners & Soap Making For Beginners

To create CP soap, prepare all of the safety tools and soap making equipment along with some freezer paper, wax paper, paper towels, and a stove. The ingredients you will need are the following: oil, skin-safe fragrance or essential oil, soap-safe colorant, sodium hydroxide lye, and distilled water. For each pound of soap you will need 11 ounces of oils. The rest will be made up of lye and water.

The following recipe will yield 3 pounds of soap. Type in the following information in SoapCalc:

Weight of Oils - 33 ounces

Water as % of Oils - 38

Super Fat % - 5

Fragrance Oz per Lb - 1

Distilled water - 12.5 oz (355.5 g)

Lye - sodium hydroxide - 4.6 oz (131.0 g)

Castor oil - 6.6 oz (186.1 g) (20%)

Coconut oil (76 degrees) - 6.6 oz (187.1 g) 20%

Palm oil - 19.8 oz (561.3 g) (60%)

The soap qualities will then be:

Hardness - 46

Cleansing - 14

Conditioning - 51

Bubbly - 32

Creamy - 50

Iodine - 51

INS - 156

The following are steps on how to create Basic Cold Process Soap. Remember to wear your safety glasses and latex gloves whenever you are about to handle lye and lye mixtures.

Essential Oils Box Set #29: Natural Homemade Cleaning Recipes for Beginners & Soap Making For Beginners

Step 1: With the shiny side up, use freezer paper to line the mold unless your mold is made of plastic.

Step 2: Set your measuring scale to ounces or grams, and place a clean empty plastic pitcher on top. After that, press the tare button to remove the pitcher's weight so that the scale will show zero. Pour water into the pitcher until you get 12.5 oz (255.5 g). Remove the pitcher and set aside.

Step 3: Put a bowl on the scale and do the same process to zero out the bowl's weight. Use a scoop or spoon to add the lye into the bowl until you get 4.6 oz (131.0 g). Remove the bowl and set aside.

Step 4: In a well-ventilated area (such as near a window or extracting fan), place the pitcher of water on a counter or sink and then very slowly add the lye to the water while stirring. Keep stirring until the lye is completely dissolved. This will make the water hot.

Step 5: Place this lye/water mixture in a secure area to cool for about 60 minutes.

Step 6: Melt and stir your palm oil on top of a stove in a stainless steel pot. It is essential to melt the oil before weighing it.

Step 7: Weight 19.8 oz (561.3 g) of the melted palm oil on your scale in a separate clean stainless steel pot. Repeat the process with castor oil for 6.6 oz (187.1 g) and coconut oil for 6.6 oz (187.1 g).

Step 8: Using a steel thermometer, check if the lye and oils have cooled to lower than 90 degrees Fahrenheit (32.22 degrees Celsius). If they are, then you can very slowly pour the lye/water mixture into the oils.

Step 9: Carefully blend the lye/water and oils together with your stainless steel spoon or blender. After they are blended well together you can add your fragrance.

Step 10: Keep stirring until you begin seeing trace. Once it gets to a Medium trace you can pour the mixture into your prepared mold. Be careful not to stir it too much such that it will reach the Thick trace; this will be very difficult to transfer into the mold.

Step 11: Cover your soap-filled mold with waxed paper or the lid of your plastic try. Let it sit for 48 hours. This will give it enough time to go through the gel stage.

Step 12: After 48 hours, you can take the soap out of the mold and transfer it to a flat surface lined with waxed paper. Let the soap air for a couple more hours before you cut them up into bars. Make sure to wear latex gloves as the lye is still active and will irritate your skin.

Step 13: Let the soap cure and completely harden before use. To test whether the lye has completely neutralized, you can do the "zap test". Very quickly tap the soap to the tip of your tongue. If the soap is just bitter (with that soapy taste), then it is good to go. If there is a slight tingle or "zap" on your tongue, it means the lye is still active and will need more time to cure.

Chapter 5 - Hot Process Soap

Hot process is a method that will produce soap instantly or with minimal cure time compared to cold compress sop. It requires you to cook the soap mixture on the stove until it fully saponifies. Set it aside and let it cool, and right after that you can start using it.

The latest instructions on how to do hot process soap is to begin with the steps in creating cold process oven process soap. The oven is also preheated to 170 degrees Fahrenheit but this time, you do not turn off the oven as you put the soap-filled mold inside of it. Let it cook at the same temperature for 4 hours. After that, you turn off the heat but do not remove the mold. Let the oven cool completely before you do so. The moment you take it out of the oven, you can cut and then use the bars immediately.

The disadvantage to using hot process is that it can be difficult to remove the soap from the mold. To make this task easier for you, what you do is to line the mold with freezer paper (shiny side up) before you pour the soap mixture into the mold. At the end of the process, the soap will not be difficult to remove from the mold.

How to Make Hot Process Soap

Prepare all of the safety and soap making equipment, along with a 2 cup measuring cup, a ceramic bowl and a stove with an oven. The following will be a basic soap recipe that will yield 17.11 oz (485.1 g) of soap.

First start with SoapCalc and type in the following details:

Weight of Oils - 11 oz

Water as % of Oils - 38

Super Fat - 8

Fragrance Oz per Lb - .7

Distilled water - 4.18 oz (118.503 g)

Lye - sodium hydroxide - 1.454 oz (41.232 g)

Beef tallow - 7.92 oz (224.532 g) (72%)

Coconut oil - 1.10 oz (31.185 g) (10%)

Castor oil - 1.10 oz (31.185 g) (10%)

Fragrance oil - .481 oz (13.640 g)

The soap qualities will then be:

Hardness - 50

Cleansing - 11

Conditioning - 48

Bubbly - 20

Creamy - 47

Iodine - 50

INS - 146

The following are steps on how to create Basic Hot Process Soap. Remember to wear your safety glasses and latex gloves whenever you are about to handle lye and lye mixtures.

Step 1: With the shiny side up, use freezer paper to line the mold unless your mold is made of plastic.

Step 2: Set your measuring scale to ounces or grams, and place the ceramic bowl on top. After that, press the tare button to remove the pitcher's weight so that the scale will show zero. Pour fragrance oil into the ceramic bowl until you get .481 oz (13.640 g). Remove the bowl and set aside.

Step 3: Put a larger bowl on the scale and push the tare button again. Weight every oil separately and add them to the stainless steel pot.

Step 4: Place the pot full of oils over medium to low heat. Allow the oils to melt completely.

Step 5: As the oils continue to be heated, put a plastic bowl on top of the scale and zero out its weight by pressing the tare button. Weight the sodium hydroxide or lye in the bowl and then set it aside.

Step 6: Put a pitcher on the scale and zero out its weight. Pour distilled water into it and weigh it, then set aside.

Step 7: After the oils are thoroughly melted, mix the lye very carefully with the water. Ensure that you are wearing your safety glasses and latex gloves. Remember to do this in a well-ventilated area as well. The lye should be sprinkled slowly into the water while stirring. Keep your face as far from the pitcher as possible because the vapors are toxic.

Step 8: Keep the pot heated over medium to low heat as you pour the lye/water mixture in with the oils. Use your immersion blender to mix all of the ingredients thoroughly

Step 9: Keep on stirring while the pot is on the stove. You will notice the soap starting to trace. Keep it heated. You will eventually notice the oils separating and floating to the top. Continue to cook until the soap mixture starts to smooth out.

Step 10: As soon as the soap mixture will turn into a mashed potato consistency, add your fragrance and stir it thoroughly. If you wish to add soap-safe colorant into your soap mixture, scoop out roughly 1 cup of the soap and add it to the bowl holding your colorant. Mix them well until the entire soap mixture is evenly tinted. Pour this back into the pot and stir until you get the effect that you want.

Step 11: Transfer the soap into your mold. Make it as smooth as you can on top. Tap the soap-filled mold onto a flat surface to force any air bubbles out. Set the mold aside to let the soap cool in room temperature.

Step 12: Once the soap is thoroughly cool, cut it into bars for use. Use a soap cutter or a long knife to do this. To cut cleanly, position yourself directly over the soap and cut straight down in one swift push.

Once you have finished making your first batch of soap, you will find that the process is not that hard. It does take a bit of patience and utmost accuracy, but the results will definitely be worth it. After you have tried any one of the recipes in this book, you can try out plenty more soap recipes that you can find on the internet or in soap making books.

Have fun with your new soap making hobby!

Conclusion

Thank you again for purchasing this book!

I hope this book was able to help you to understand what you need in order to start making natural homemade soap at home.

The next step is to start processing your first batch of soap.

Finally, if you enjoyed this book, please take the time to share your thoughts and post a review on Amazon. We do our best to reach out to readers and provide the best value we can. Your positive review will help us achieve that. It'd be greatly appreciated!

Thank you and good luck!

Check Out My Other Books

Below you'll find some of my other popular books that are popular on Amazon and Kindle as well. Simply click on the links below to check them out. Alternatively, you can visit my author page on Amazon to see other work done by me.

Coconut Oil for Easy Weight Loss

http://amzn.to/1i5f45p

Carrier Oils For Beginners

http://amzn.to/1sbqUQP

Natural Homemade Cleaning Recipes For Beginners

http://amzn.to/1izDB2m

Essential Oils & Aromatherapy

http://amzn.to/1ouuZTx

Superfoods that Kickstart Your Weight Loss

http://amzn.to/1eyHdku

The Best Secrets Of Natural Remedies

http://amzn.to/1gmHd7y

The Hypothyroidism Handbook

http://amzn.to/1emWfyR

Essential Oils Box Set #29: Natural Homemade Cleaning Recipes for Beginners & Soap Making For Beginners

The Hyperthyroidism Handbook

http://amzn.to/1kqLQCp

Essential Oils & Weight Loss For Beginners

http://amzn.to/Q83bFp

Top Essential Oil Recipes

http://amzn.to/1lSrhSC

Soap Making For Beginners

http://amzn.to/1fkmYwr

Body Butters For Beginners

http://amzn.to/1fWjwJe

Apple Cider Vinegar For Beginners

http://amzn.to/1joDzX2

Homemade Body Scrubs & Masks For Beginners

http://amzn.to/1jjLRIO

Essential Oils Box Set #1 (Weight Loss + Essential Oil Recipes

http://amzn.to/1qlYWWP

Essential Oils Box Set #2 (Weight Loss + Essential Oil & Aromatherapy

http://amzn.to/1qlYWWP

Essential Oils Box Set #29: Natural Homemade Cleaning Recipes for Beginners & Soap Making For Beginners

Essential Oils Box Set #3 Coconut Oil + Apple Cider Vinegar

http://amzn.to/1oIFZJw

Essential Oils Box Set #4 Body Butters & Top Essential Oil Recipes

http://amzn.to/1jSxURJ

Essential Oils Box Set #5 Soap Making & Homemade Body Scrubs

http://amzn.to/RAvJYo

Essential Oils Box Set #6 Body Butters & Body Scrubs

http://amzn.to/RAvSel

Essential Oils Box Set #7 Top Essential Oils & Best Kept Secrets Of Natural Remedies

http://amzn.to/1gvsRCq

Essential Oils Box Set #11 Carrier Oils for Beginners & Coconut Oil for Easy Weight Loss

http://amzn.to/1nHfy6X

Essential Oils Box Set #12 Essential Oils Weight Loss & Essential Oils Aromatherapy & Natural Homemade Cleaning Supplies & Top Essential Oil Recipes & Carrier Oils
http://amzn.to/1nHfy6X

Essential Oils Box Set #13 Superfoods & Essential Weight Loss & Essential Aromatherapy & Body Butters & Soap Making
http://amzn.to/1nUds6v

Essential Oils Box Set #29: Natural Homemade Cleaning Recipes for Beginners & Soap Making For Beginners

Essential Oils Box Set #14 Weight Loss & Apple Cider Vinegar & Body Butters & Homemade Body Scrubs & Coconut Oil for Beginners

http://amzn.to/1i1qYOd

If the links do not work, for whatever reason, you can simply search for these titles on the Amazon website to find them.

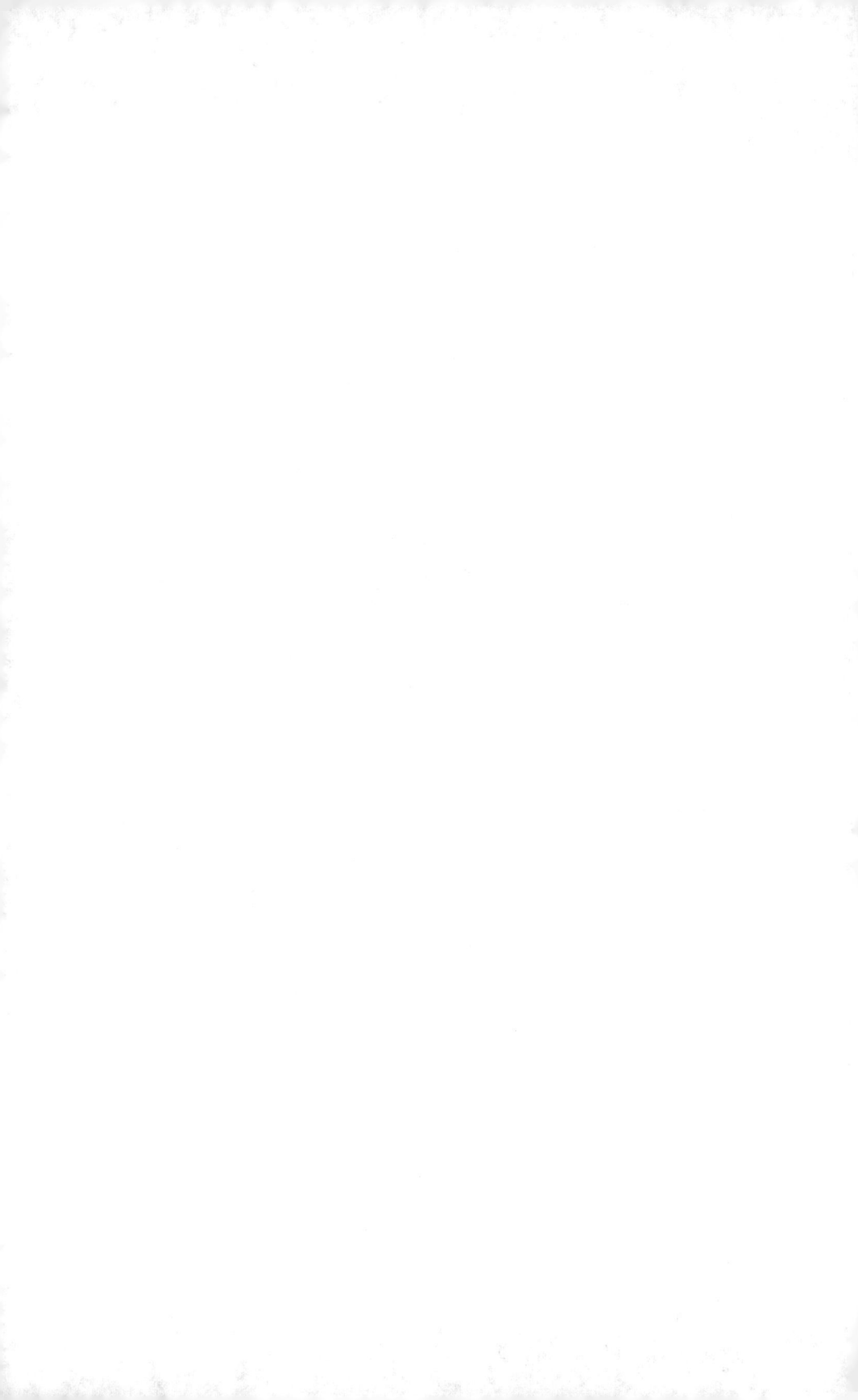

www.ingramcontent.com/pod-product-compliance
Lightning Source LLC
Chambersburg PA
CBHW070609290526
45790CB00002B/844